a morning cup of massage™

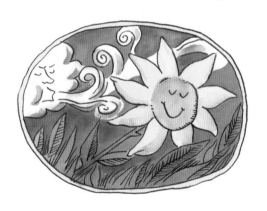

The publisher and author cannot be held responsible for injury, mishap, or damages incurred during the performance of the exercises in this book. The author recommends consultation with a healthcare professional before beginning this or any other exercise program.

"A Morning Cup of" is a trademark of Crane Hill Publishers, Inc.

Published by Crane Hill Publishers
www.cranehill.com

Printed in China

Library of Congress Cataloging-in-Publication Data

Bright-Fey, Kim.
  A morning cup of massage : one 15-minute routine for a lifetime of energy and harmony / Kim Bright-Fey.
      p. cm.
   ISBN-13: 978-1-57587-237-7
   ISBN-10: 1-57587-237-4
   1. Massage. 2. Self-care, Health. I. Title.
   RA780.5B73 2005
   615.8'22--dc22
                                2005019018

Meridian diagram on page 16 from The Association For Meridian & Energy Therapies. http://TheAMT.com.

a morning cup of massage™

one 15-minute routine for a lifetime of energy & harmony

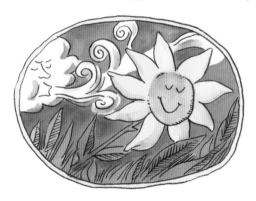

kim bright-fey, p.t.

CRANE HILL
PUBLISHERS

Acknowledgments

Thank you to John Bright-Fey, my husband, who taught me everything I know about Traditional Chinese Medicine. John created the *New Forest*® Qi massage routine based on his extensive knowledge. I have used this routine for many years to help myself and to help my clients. It works! Thank you, John! Without you, this book would not have been possible.

Thank you to all at Crane Hill Publishers for showing an interest in this work and making it become a reality.

Contents

Foreword

Chinese therapeutic massage is one of the oldest medical interventions in recorded history. It was first described in the Huang Di Nei Jing (*Yellow Emperor's Classic of Internal Medicine*), written circa 2600 BCE. Think about that for a moment; Chinese massage has been field-tested by real people in real-life situations for more than forty-six thousand years!

I can think of no one better than Kim Bright-Fey to present the wonders of Qi massage. We have worked together as professionals for nearly two decades. Kim has the rare ability to effortlessly bridge the gap between the Eastern and Western medical models. She intuitively joins science with sensitivity and empowers each of her clients to create, on their own, a more harmonious life. Now, it's your turn.

Qi massage is the result of a unique health and wellness perspective that sees great beauty, sophisticated design, and immense wisdom in the human body. *A Morning Cup of Massage* will show you how to access that wisdom, understand the design, and bask in the beauty of yourself. It is the perfect guide to a new world of physical, mental, and spiritual well being.

John Bright-Fey
Tai Chi Grand Master and
author of *A Morning Cup of Tai Chi*,
A Morning Cup of Meditation,
and *A Morning Cup of Qigong*

The Magic of Massage

As a physical therapist, I have spent nearly twenty years using my hands to help individuals feel better and function at their best. Some of my clients tell me that my hands are magic. Your hands can be magic, too! You simply need to train them to be sensitive and to respond in a natural and instinctive way. This book will show you how.

In a simple 15-minute self-massage routine that you can do in the comfort of your own home, you will learn how to rub and massage your body along the energy pathways used by acupuncturists. You will learn a Qi massage to cultivate the smooth and unrestricted flow of energy throughout your entire system. You will feel relaxed and energized at the same time.

This book begins with some basic but important information about massage and Traditional Chinese Medicine. I recommend reading these sections before you begin your self-massage routine. Understanding how and why massage works will give you the best results.

I have also included massage techniques that you can share with a friend. You will find these exercises toward the end of the book in the section titled An Extra Sip. As with all the books in the Morning Cup series, there is an audio CD inserted in the back cover. Once you are familiar with the routine, put the disc into your CD player and follow along.

It's time to learn how to make your hands MAGIC! Let's begin.

Kim Bright-Fey
Birmingham, Alabama
Fall 2005

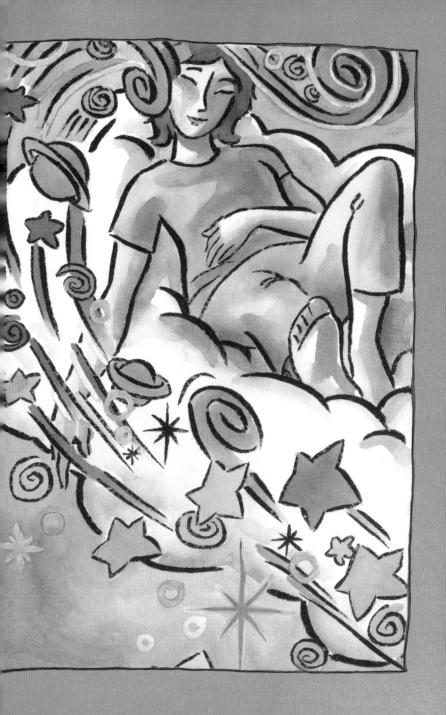

The Benefits of Massage

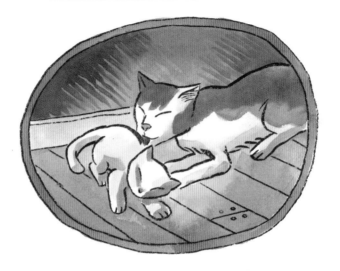

Everyone has experienced the benefits of massage, even you! When you wake in the morning, you rub your eyes to see more clearly. When you are cold, you rub your arms to generate heat. When you bump your leg, you rub it to make it feel better. Massage is a natural approach to health and wellness.

In the past decade, massage has become one of the most popular forms of complementary care. Studies show that more people than ever are seeking massage to manage stress and relieve pain. The American Massage Therapy Association reports that consumers spend nearly $4 billion a year on visits to massage therapists.

Massage can't cure everything that ails you, but it certainly feels good!

What you can expect from massage:

Physical Benefits
- Improves circulation and blood flow
- Reduces muscle spasm and pain
- Boosts the immune systems and speeds healing
- Improves mobility and promotes flexibility

Mental/Emotional Benefits
- Reduces mental stress and anxiety
- Increases awareness of bodymind connection
- Improves sense of well being

The Risks of Massage

Massage is generally very safe and has very few risks. However, massage is not for everyone. It is always a good idea to talk to your doctor before engaging in any new health or exercise regimen. This is especially true if you have any of the following conditions:

- Open wounds, burns, or skin ailments
- Deep vein thrombosis, phlebitis, or edema
- Lymphedema or cancer
- Heart condition
- Severe osteoporosis
- Recent injury, such as strain, sprain, or fracture
- Pregnancy

Injuries from massage are rare and are most often caused by too much pressure. If too much pressure is being used, tell your therapist. Don't be shy. Your therapist will gladly adjust his or her technique to make it more comfortable for you. The techniques in this book use very light pressure and are designed to be safe and effective for almost anyone.

Massage Professionals

As the popularity of massage has grown, the choices available to you have expanded exponentially. To make the best decision when seeking the services of a massage professional, ask yourself the reason that you want to get a massage.

Do You Need Relief from Everyday Stress and Tension?

If you suffer from muscular aches and pains caused by stress and overwork, you might want to see a massage therapist. Massage therapists are either licensed or certified. The requirements are different from state to state. Most massage therapists have two years of extensive training in manual therapy or massage techniques. Massage therapists are experts in providing hands-on care. The effects of a good massage can last for weeks and often can interrupt the cycle of muscle spasms and pain for long-term relief.

Do You Need Pain Relief Caused by a Specific Condition?

If you suffer from a condition such as arthritis, fibromyalgia, sciatica, or chronic back pain, you might want to see a physical therapist (PT). Physical therapists are licensed medical professionals and have completed six years of education. They are trained to diagnose the underlying cause of your pain and communicate with your physician about your treatment and progress. Most chronic pain conditions are worsened by poor posture habits and muscle imbalances. In addition to massage, a PT will teach you exercises to stretch muscles that are tight and strengthen muscles that are weak. The goal of a physical therapist is to provide a long-term solution to your pain.

Types of Massage

There are many different types of massage. Some of the most common include:

- **Swedish Massage.** Long gliding strokes are combined with gentle kneading and compression techniques to provide an overall sense of relaxation. This is the most common type of massage in the U.S.

- **Deep Tissue Massage.** As the term implies, the focus of this type of massage is on your muscles and soft tissues that lie deep beneath your skin. Rolfing, Trager, and trigger-point therapy are all forms of deep tissue massage. Caution must be used to avoid injury from overpressure.

- **Sports Massage.** Specific muscle groups are targeted to improve athletic performance. Massage prior to an athletic event can release unwanted tension and improve flexibility. Massage after an event has been shown to reduce post-exercise soreness.

- **Asian Massage.** The goal of an Asian-based method is to balance your body's energy, or Qi (pronounced chee). Light stroking and pressure applied at specific points are common treatment techniques. Acupressure, Shiatsu, and Reiki are all forms of Asian massage and are based on the principles of Traditional Chinese Medicine. The routine found in this book is an Asian-based massage.

Chinese Medicine and Massage

A central concept of Chinese Medicine is that good health depends on the smooth and unrestricted flow of Qi, or vital life-force energy. Herbs, acupuncture, exercise (like Tai Chi), and massage are used to facilitate the healthy flow of Qi.

Qi travels along very specific pathways called meridians. Take a moment to look at the diagram on page 16 showing the meridians running through your body. Notice that you have meridians, or energy pathways, on your head, torso, arms, and legs. Your body is covered with these invisible pathways! Most lie close to the surface of your skin, but many travel deep into your tissues and vital body organs.

To understand the flow of Qi and why it is important to your health, consider this analogy: Pretend that the meridian pathways are highways. A properly functioning highway has cars and trucks moving freely at the designated speed limit. Sometimes there are problems.

Perhaps one lane is closed for construction. The traffic slows and can bottleneck at that spot. Sometimes there aren't many cars on the road. You might be tempted to drive too fast or you might drive too slow, getting lost in your own thoughts. Often times, there are too many cars and trucks on the road. The traffic is congested and flows at erratic speeds.

Highways need cars and trucks flowing freely. Your meridians need Qi flowing freely. Blockages and construction cause problems. Too much or too little traffic/Qi flow can cause different problems. Highways and meridians need smooth and unrestricted flow to function properly.

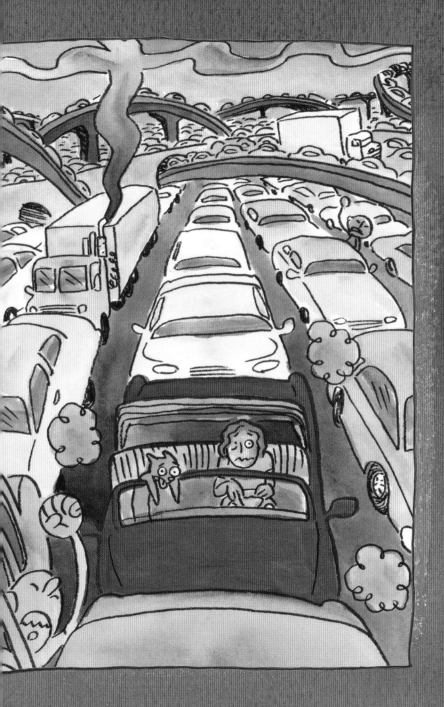

Meridian Pathways

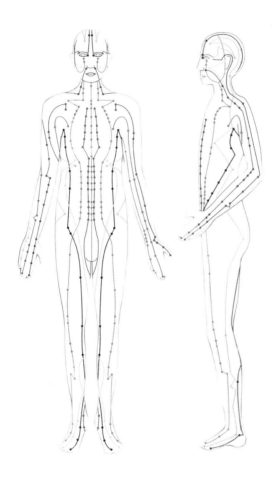

Qi Massage: Cultivating Balance

Cultivation is a term that is frequently used in Chinese medicine. I like it because I am a gardener. I love to work in my yard and I can relate to the importance of cultivating the soil. If I don't take the time and effort to cultivate the soil, my plants suffer. When I prepare the soil properly, my plants thrive.

The Qi massage routine in this book is designed to help you cultivate a balance of energy flowing through your bodymind. I blend the two words together because in reality, they are one. Your body and mind cannot be separated. The energy flowing through your muscles, skin, and vital body organs is connected to your thoughts and attitudes.

Modern science now proves that laughter really is good medicine, and a daily Qi massage is a great way to get in shape and stay healthy. In fact, you will notice an improvement if you perform your massage routine as little as 2-3 times each week. Massaging yourself provides the same benefit as receiving a massage from someone else.

The 15-minute Qi massage in this book will:
• Reduce your pain and tension
• Reduce your stress and anxiety
• Improve your circulation and blood flow
• Boost your immune system and promote healing
• Improve your awareness of your body

And, IT'S FREE!
Self-applied massage takes only a few minutes out of your busy day!

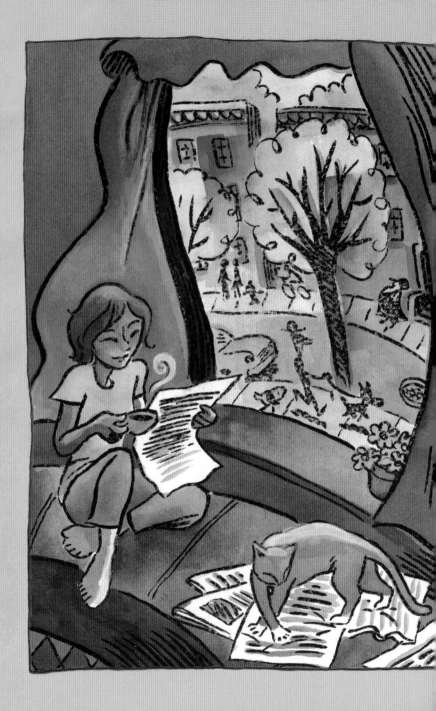

The Routine

New Forest® Qi Massage

Qi massage is similar to other types of massage in that you will be using long gliding strokes and the application of pressure to specific points on your body. It is different from other types of massage because you will not focus on specific muscle groups. Each technique you will perform is designed to address the flow of Qi along your meridian pathways. It is a holistic approach.

In the *Extra Attention* boxes, you will find suggestions and additional information about each technique. The audio CD in the back of the book will lead you through the routine in about 15 minutes. For best results, please read the book first and get familiar with each technique before using the CD.

You can perform New Forest Qi massage at any time of the day, but doing it before or after your morning cup will help you establish a healthy routine. If you start your day with Tai Chi, or other fitness program, perform your massage at the end of your exercise session.

Follow These Other Tips for Best Results:
- Wear loose, comfortable clothing that allows you to move freely. You will need to be barefoot for the foot massage.
- Remove your jewelry.
- Wash and moisturize your hands. Trim or file your fingernails so they have smooth edges. Shorter fingernails are better for massage than long ones.
- Create a pleasant environment. Play soft, soothing music. Light your favorite scented candle.
- Do not perform your Qi massage immediately after a heavy meal.
- Qi massage should never cause pain. If a movement is painful, stop doing it. Try making the movement softer and smaller. If that doesn't help, skip to the next exercise.
- Sit down and rest if you feel dizzy or lightheaded. Do not continue with the program until these feelings pass. If they don't pass within a couple of minutes, consult your doctor.

Some Advice on Breathing:
- Keep your breath natural and relaxed during massage. Listening to your body's natural rhythm of breath has a very calming effect on your central nervous system. Whenever possible, breathe in and out through your nose and relax your lower abdomen to allow deeper breathing. Never hold or restrict your breathing.

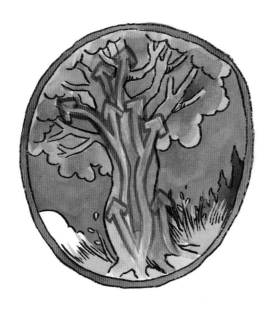

Part One: Activate and Stimulate

Your Qi massage routine begins with a full body rub designed to activate and stimulate the Qi energy that runs through your meridians. Once you learn the sequence, your full body rub takes only a couple of minutes. This part of the routine is called an "air bath" in Chinese medicine. As you perform the massaging motions, suggest to yourself that you are wiping away stress, tension, and pockets of stagnant energy. The full body rub is like the pre-wash cycle on your washing machine, and prepares you for precise massage techniques, but can also be used as a 2-3 minute stress break in the middle of your busy day.

Activate Your Hands

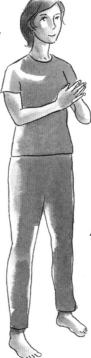

1. Stand comfortably with your knees bent slightly.

2. Clap your hands together.

3. Rub them back and forth.

4. Rub them all over: fronts, backs, and in between your fingers. Rub, rub, rub!

Extra Attention

Acupuncture meridians begin and end in your hands and feet. Clapping your hands together and rubbing them back and forth stimulates your Qi-energy and generates heat, even if you can't feel it. Don't be disappointed if your hands don't get warm. You are activating your Qi-energy and preparing your hands for your energetic massage.

Activate Your Arms

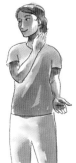

1. Place your right palm below your left ear.

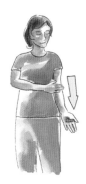

2. Turn your left hand so it is palm up. Slide your right hand down your left arm. Use a light and gentle pressure as if you were rubbing on suntan lotion.

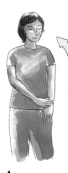

3. Turn your left palm down, and slide your arm up, returning to just below your ear.

4. Do 3 times on your left arm and 3 times on your right arm.

Extra Attention

Remember that you are massaging your energy pathways. Your light touch stimulates the Qi energy to flow freely through the meridians that are in your arms. In time, you will feel the energy moving down your arm when your palm is up and up your arm when your palm is facing down. Pressing too hard causes the pathways to collapse, like a roadblock. Be patient. Remember, lighter is better.

Activate Your Back

1. Place your palms on your low back. Rub your low back all over. Rub, rub, rub.

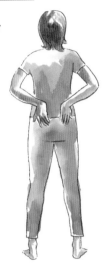

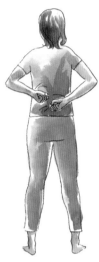

2. Make your hands into fists. Gently pound up and down beside your spine. Lightly beat, beat, beat.

Extra Attention

Most of us carry tension in our low back. Back pain is extremely common in our over-stressed modern culture. Touching and rubbing your low back will help you bring your attention and awareness to this part of your body. As you become more aware of your low back, you will be able to identify the tension early, as it begins to develop. Early identification of tension is a key to preventing chronic low back pain. Pay attention to how your back feels today; compare it to how it felt yesterday.

Activate Your Legs

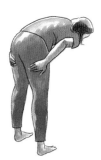

1. Place your palms on your low back.

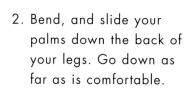

2. Bend, and slide your palms down the back of your legs. Go down as far as is comfortable.

3. Bring your palms to the inside of your legs. Slide up, traveling to the tops of your thighs, and then to your waist.

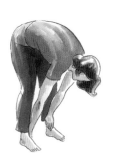

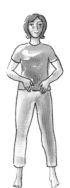

4. Repeat 2 times.

Extra Attention

Bending over creates tremendous pressure in the spine. If you have problems, like a herniated disc or osteoporosis, use caution. If sliding your hands below your knees is uncomfortable or unsafe for you, use your imagination to visualize the movement. Visualization affects your body's energy the same way as physical contact, and you will get better at it with practice. You can also do this movement sitting in a chair and get the same benefit.

Activate Your Belly

1. Place your palms on your belly.

2. Use light pressure to circle and rub all over your abdomen.

3. Let each hand work independently. Rub, rub, rub.

4. Circle and rub.

5. Get all over; don't miss a spot!

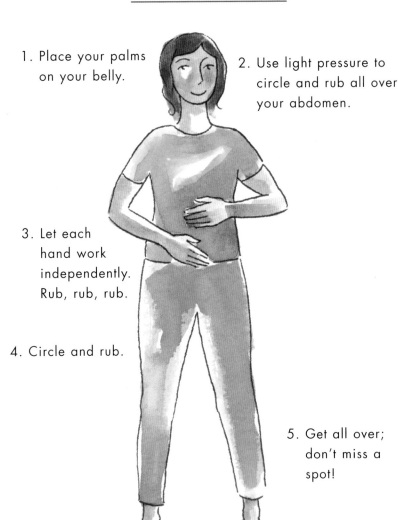

Activate Your Head and Scalp

1. Make light fists with your hands.

2. Gently scrub your scalp. Cover every inch as if you were shampooing your head with your knuckles. Rub, rub, rub.

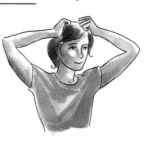

3. Open your hands and gently rub your ears with your fingers. Rub them all over.

4. Gently pinch your ears between your thumb and first finger.

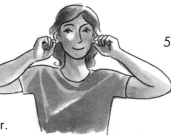

5. Softly squeeze and pinch the upper and lower lobes.

Extra Attention

Your ears are considered a link to your whole body in Traditional Chinese Medicine. It is theorized that the ear contains a miniature version of your whole self. If you find a particular spot on your ear that is tender, spend a few moments gently squeezing and releasing that area. It may indicate an energy blockage somewhere else in your body. Massaging the ear will have a positive effect on your whole body.

Finishing the Full Body Rub

Do this exercise to end your "air bath." It will help relax you and center your healing energy.

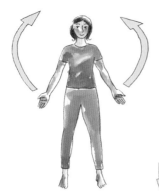

1. Stand with your feet parallel and shoulder width apart.

2. Lift your arms out and up, bringing your hands to the top of your head.

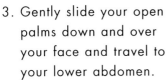
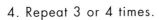
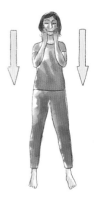

3. Gently slide your open palms down and over your face and travel to your lower abdomen.

4. Repeat 3 or 4 times.

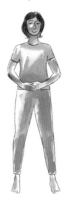

5. Finish by placing your hands over your lower abdomen. If you are female, place your right hand on top of your left. If you are male, place your left hand on top of your right. Stand quietly for a moment before moving on to the next section.

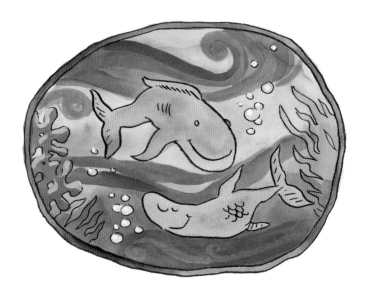

Part Two: Refine and Tonify

Sit comfortably in a chair. It is time to zero in on specific parts of your body. These techniques are designed to refine and tonify your Qi. Tonify is a term commonly used in Chinese medicine. It basically means that you are balancing the tone of your energy. Qi massage will help increase energy flow in areas that have too little Qi and reduce energy flow in areas that have too much Qi. The goal of Qi massage is for Qi to run smoothly and evenly throughout your entire system.

Let's begin at the top and work our way down!

Head Massage

Activate your hands by rubbing them together.

Pound Your Neck

1. Make a gentle fist with your right hand.

2. Grab your right upper arm with your left hand, and tilt your head to the right.

3. Gently pound along the left side of your neck and travel to your shoulder.

4. Lightly pound up and down along this stretch of muscle for a count of ten.

5. Repeat on the other side.

Extra Attention

Muscular tension is common in the neck and shoulders. Many of us are so tense that we carry our shoulders up around our ears. Try this exercise to help identify tension and learn how to consciously relax. 1. Lift your shoulders toward your ears in a shrugging-motion. 2. Slowly allow your shoulders to drop. Lengthen your neck by stretching up with the top of your head. Gently pound the muscles as instructed in this exercise and suggest to yourself that you will allow your shoulders to stay down and relaxed.

Circling the Eye

1. Place the pads of your index fingers together at the inside corners of your eyebrows.

2. Separate, and gently and slowly circle around your eyes.

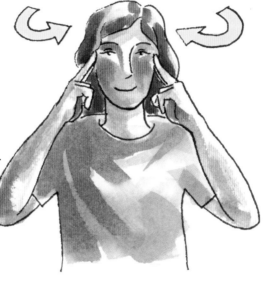

3. Stay on the bony part that surrounds your eyes.

4. Circle gently 5-10 times.

Extra Attention

The skin around your eye is very thin and delicate. Your touch should be so light that it does not stretch or distort the skin. Gently skim over the surface of your skin. The motion will bring your attention and awareness to the muscles that surround your eye. Notice the tension that you accumulate when you squint your eyes. Allow your facial muscles to relax. This exercise will help reduce the appearance of forehead creases and crow's feet.

Nasal Flare

1. Place the pads of your index fingers at the bottom of your nasal flare.

2. Without lifting your fingers, press in lightly and massage.

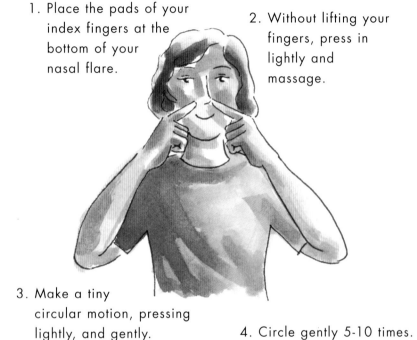

3. Make a tiny circular motion, pressing lightly, and gently.

4. Circle gently 5-10 times.

Extra Attention

The acupoint located in this spot is very important in regulating your internal organs. Gentle pressure and massage will help relax your stomach and promote circulation through your guts and viscera.

Corner Of Eye

1. Place the pads of your index fingers at the outside corner of your eye. Be sure to stay on the bony part and avoid your temple.

2. Without lifting your fingers, lightly press and massage.

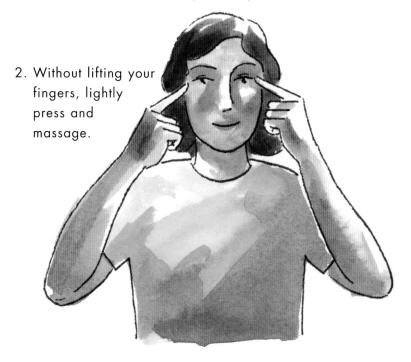

3. Make a tiny circular motion, pressing lightly, being gentle!

4. Circle gently 5-10 times.

Sinus Massage

1. Pinch the bridge of your nose with one hand.

2. With the other, gently, but firmly grasp your forehead with your thumb and first two fingers. Make sure to avoid your temples!

3. Move your hands in opposite directions from side to side.

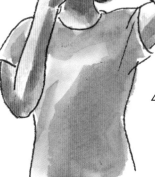

4. Using firm but gentle pressure, rock your hands back and forth.

5. Repeat 5-10 times.

Extra Attention

This technique requires a bit of grip strength. Be forceful but gentle. Never do anything that causes pain. As always, experiment with the hand placement and technique to find what feels most comfortable for you. This technique is wonderful to reduce the pain from sinus pressure and sinus headaches. Allow your hands and arms to relax fully before moving on to the next exercise.

Jaw Hinge

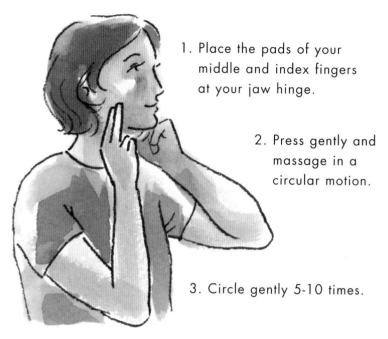

1. Place the pads of your middle and index fingers at your jaw hinge.

2. Press gently and massage in a circular motion.

3. Circle gently 5-10 times.

Extra Attention

Experiment with the amount of pressure that you can tolerate on your jaw muscles. These are the thickest and perhaps strongest muscles in your face. Feel free to press a bit more firmly with this exercise. Many of us clench our jaws or grind our teeth without even knowing it. Tension in the jaw muscles can cause jaw pain and headaches. Use this technique to monitor your tension level and help you learn to identify when you are unconsciously clenching and grinding your teeth.

Head Drumming

1. Place your hands over your ears so that your fingers are at the back of your head. Experiment to find a comfortable position.

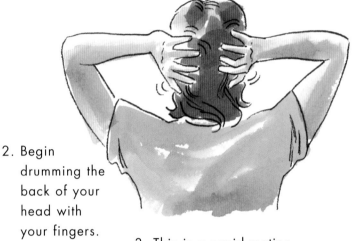

2. Begin drumming the back of your head with your fingers.

3. This is a rapid motion. Drum, drum, drum!

4. Continue for 10 seconds.

Extra Attention

Tension headaches are typically due to muscular spasms and tension in the muscles at the base of your skull. This is a great technique to use at work or after a long period of sitting. The drumming motion provides gentle vibration that causes the muscles to relax. Energy that is trapped in this area will be able to flow more evenly and you will feel better.

Head Rub

1. Make gentle fists and use your knuckles to rub every inch of your scalp.

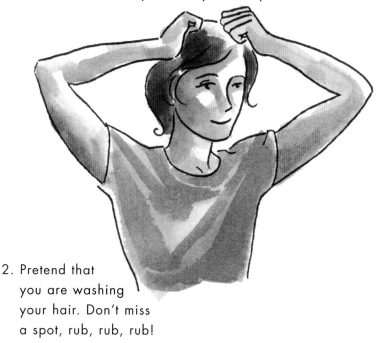

2. Pretend that you are washing your hair. Don't miss a spot, rub, rub, rub!

Extra Attention

You have important acupoints on the top and back of your head. In Traditional Chinese Medicine they are considered energy gathering points. Rubbing the scalp stimulates these points and promotes the smooth and unrestricted flow of Qi energy. Use this technique to clear your thinking and energize your body.

Abdomen Massage

Belly Circle 1

1. If you are female, place your right hand over your left. If you are male, place your left hand over your right.

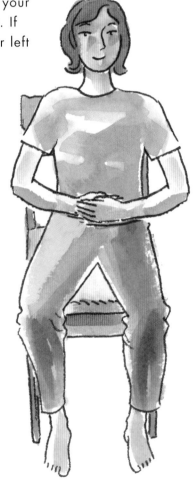

2. Using your palm and light pressure, make one large clockwise circle around your abdomen.

3. Return to your start position. Repeat 5-10 times.

Belly Circle 2

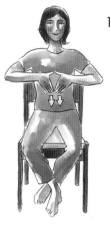

1. Place the pads of your fingers at the uppermost part of your belly, between your ribs.

2. Slide down your center line to your pubic bone.

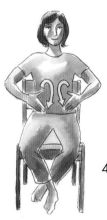

3. Separate your hands, and come up the sides of your belly, returning to your start position.

4. Do 5-10 repetitions.

Extra Attention

Many of us carry tension in our abdomen without even knowing it. Tension causes tightness, and this restricts the flow of energy and overall circulation. More than 20% of Americans suffer from irritable bowel syndrome and constipation. The 3-part Belly Circling Routine can help reduce tension in the abdominal muscles as well as the guts and viscera. In time and with practice, you will become aware of abdominal tension and tightness and learn how to keep this area relaxed.

Belly Circle 3

1. Locate the spot on your center line that is halfway between your navel and the bottom of your breastbone (A).

2. Using the pads of your fingers and gentle pressure, circle clockwise around this spot 5-10 times.

3. Move down and repeat around your belly button (B), circling 5-10 times.

4. Slide down to the spot that is halfway between your navel and pubic bone (C).

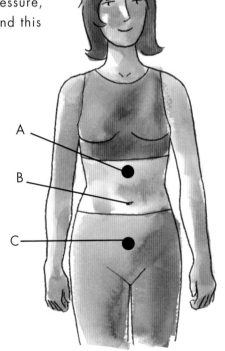

5. Remembering to use the pads of your fingers and gentle pressure, circle clockwise around this spot 5-10 times.

Hand Massage

Activate Your Hands

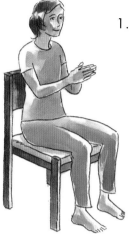

1. Rub your hands together. Back and forth, back and forth.

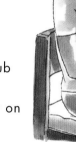

2. Take one hand and rub the back of the other. Rub, rub, rub. Repeat on the other side.

Extra Attention

In massage, your hands are your tools. Rubbing your hands together briskly not only activates your Qi, it also clears any blockages or pockets of stagnation that may have accumulated in the previous exercise. Take the time to clear your hands and reactivate!

Center of Palm

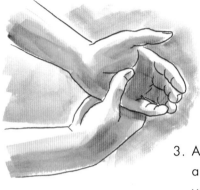

1. Place the thumb of one hand in the palm of the other.

2. As you inhale, do nothing.

3. As you exhale, gently press and massage the center of your palm.

4. Repeat 3-5 times on each hand.

Extra Attention

There is a very important acupoint in the center of your palm. In Traditional Chinese Medicine it is called the Small Star and is considered an energy gathering point. You tend to gather more energy as you inhale. It is important to press on this spot only when you are breathing out, or exhaling. Allow your thumb to rest gently against your palm as you inhale, but don't press! Pressure on the Small Star while breathing in is similar to holding a door closed. You want to leave the door open so energy can gather and be absorbed.

Tiger's Mouth

1. Place the pad of your thumb on the Tiger's Mouth area of your other hand.

2. Use your index finger and thumb to gently hold this soft part of your hand.

3. As you inhale, do nothing.

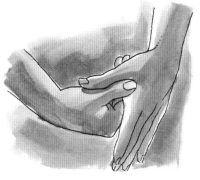

4. As you exhale, use your thumb and index finger to apply a gentle combination of squeezing and massaging.

5. Repeat 3-5 times on each hand.

Extra Attention

The Tiger's Mouth is a very important acupoint. Massaging this spot can help calm the stomach, reduce stomach acid, and get rid of headaches. According to Traditional Chinese Medicine, headaches are often caused by problems in the stomach. If you suffer from headaches or acid stomach, massage your Tiger's Mouth periodically throughout the day.

Knuckle Wiggle

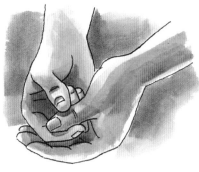

1. Gently grasp the first knuckle of your thumb.

2. Use a light pinching grip with the fingertips of your other hand.

3. As you inhale, simply hold the knuckle. As you exhale, gently twist it back and forth.

4. Move to your index finger and lightly pinch the first knuckle. As you inhale, simply hold. As you exhale, gently twist it back and forth.

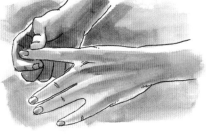

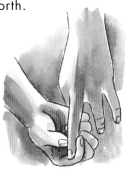

5. Move to your middle finger. Inhale and lightly grasp. Exhale and gently twist.

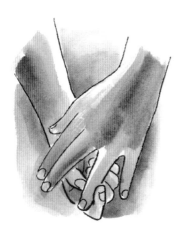

6. Move to your Ring Finger. Inhale and lightly grasp. Exhale and gently twist.

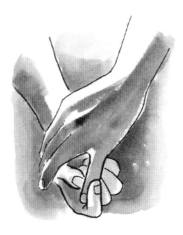

7. Move to your pinky Finger. Inhale and lightly grasp. Exhale and gently twist.

8. Repeat on the other hand.

Extra Attention

Be gentle with yourself as you wiggle your knuckles. Your touch should be light and not cause any pain or discomfort. You are simply making contact and activating each finger. As the illustration on page 48 shows, each finger corresponds to an internal organ by way of a meridian, or energetic pathway. This contact will stimulate the meridian and promote the free and unrestricted flow of Qi energy. Avoid the practice of popping or cracking your knuckles. It can become habit forming and is an unhealthy practice.

Open - Close Hands

1. Rest your hands comfortably on your thighs palm up.

2. Gradually make fists with your hands as you feel yourself inhaling.

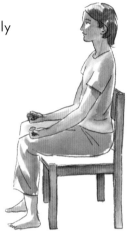

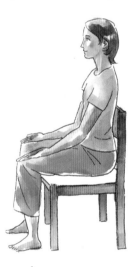

3. As you exhale, slowly open your palms and stretch the fingers outward.

4. Inhale, and slowly make fists. Exhale and open and stretch.

5. Repeat for 3-5 breaths.

Extra Attention

Allow your breath to be natural. Do not force it to be any different than it was a moment ago. Find the rhythm of your breath and match your movement to it. Learning to listen to your natural rhythm takes time. It is a skill that gets better with practice.

Thumb Hold

1. Make a gentle fist with your thumb on the inside.

2. Wrap your fingers over your thumbs and sit quietly for a moment.

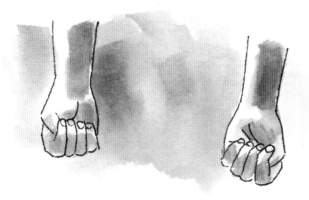

3. Use this time to feel the natural rhythm of your breath.

4. Relax.

5. Gently hold your thumb for 3-5 breaths.

Hand - Organ Correspondents

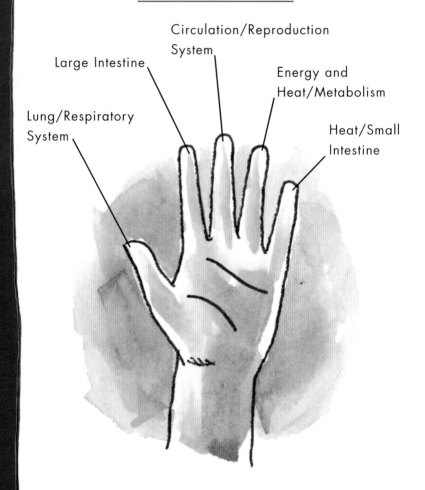

Foot - Organ Correspondents

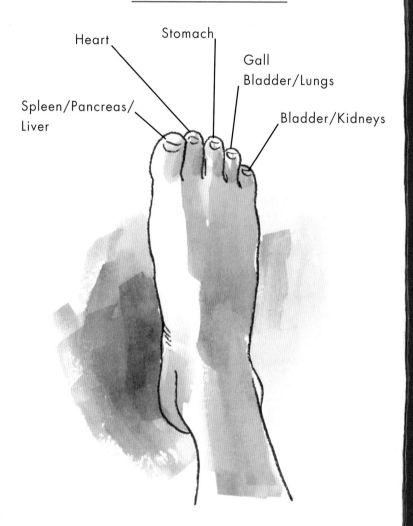

Foot Massage

Perform the entire foot massage on one foot and then repeat on the other side.

Activate Your Hands and Feet

1. Cross your legs so you can reach your right foot comfortably.

2. Using one hand to support your leg and one hand to rub, rub your foot all over.

3. Rub back and forth all over the bottom, all over the top, rub, rub, rub.

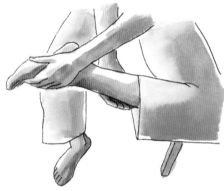

Extra Attention

Meridians, or energy pathways, begin and end in your hands and feet. Rubbing the top and bottom of your foot excites the Qi energy and generates heat, even if you don't feel it. An alternative way to rub your feet is to slide them back and forth on the floor while you are sitting. To get the top of your feet, use one foot to rub the other!

Center of Foot

1. Place the pad of your thumb in the center of your foot, just below the ball. Use whichever hand is most comfortable for you.

2. As you inhale, do nothing.

3. As you exhale, gently press and massage this spot.

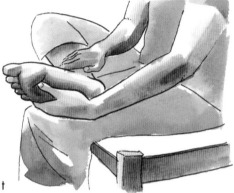

4. Inhale, maintain light contact. Exhale, press, and massage.

5. Repeat 3-5 times.

Extra Attention

There is a very important acupoint in the center of your foot. In Traditional Chinese Medicine it is called the Small Star and is considered an energy gathering point. You tend to gather more energy as you inhale. It is important to press on this spot only when you are breathing out, or exhaling. Allow your thumb to rest gently against your foot as you inhale, but don't press! Pressure on the Small Star while breathing in is similar to holding a door closed. You want to leave the door open so energy can gather and be absorbed.

Heel Massage

1. Cup your heel with your palm.

2. Anchor and support your foot with the other hand.

3. Massage your entire heel. Gently squeeze and release.

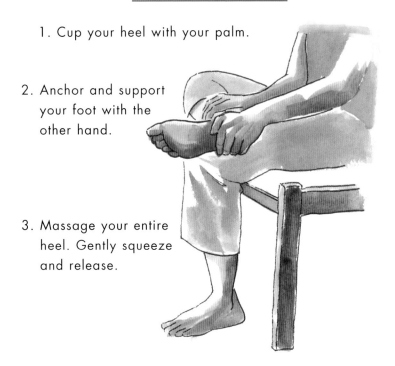

4. Squeeze and twist. Work all over the heel, massaging firmly but gently.

Extra Attention

Many people suffer from heel pain. Massaging the heel will increase blood and energy flow to this area and promote healing. If you have heel pain first thing in the morning, try doing this technique before you get out of bed. Add a few Point and Flex stretches found on page 55, and you might solve your problem!

Knuckle Wiggle

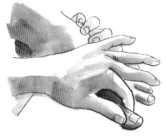

1. Gently grasp the first knuckle of your big toe. Use a light pinching grip.

2. As you inhale, simply hold the knuckle. As you exhale, gently twist it back and forth.

3. Move to your second toe, gently pinch the top knuckle.

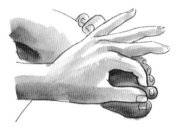

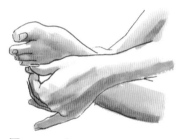

4. Keep going until you have done all of your toes.

Extra Attention

Be gentle with yourself as you wiggle your knuckles. Your touch should be light and not cause any pain or discomfort. You are simply making contact and activating each toe. As the illustration on page 49 shows, each toe corresponds to an internal organ by way of a meridian, or energetic pathway. This contact will stimulate the meridian and promote the free and unrestricted flow of Qi energy.

Foot Pounding

1. Make a loose fist and gently pound the bottom of your foot.

2. Use your other hand to anchor and support. Pound, pound, pound.

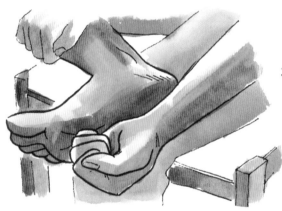

3. Move all around, pounding gently.

4. Get the heel, the arch, the ball, and your toes...pound all over!

Extra Attention

The 'pounding' technique requires a bit of practice. Most people have a tendency to tense their whole body when they make a fist. Let your arm relax as you pound your foot. Try to use as little muscular effort as possible. Feel your hand rebound off of your foot as if bouncing off a drum.

Point and Flex

1. Anchor your foot with one hand and use the other to bend the toes back and forth.

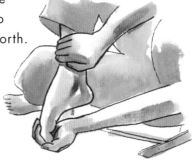

2. Inhale, and bend the toes over to stretch the top of your foot.

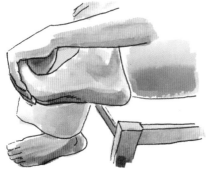

3. Exhale, and curl the toes back to stretch the arch.

4. Repeat 3-5 times.

Extra Attention

This exercise is similar to the Open-Close technique for your hand on page 46. The difference is that you allow your foot to remain passive during the technique. Let your hand do the work; Point and Flex. You are stretching the meridians on the top and then on the bottom of your foot. The result is a massaging, pumping action that promotes the smooth and unrestricted flow of Qi energy.

Foot Stomp

1. Put your foot on the floor and stomp it gently a few times. Stomp, stomp, stomp!

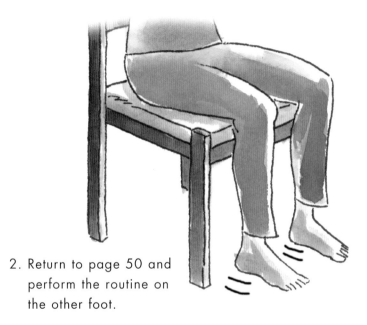

2. Return to page 50 and perform the routine on the other foot.

Extra Attention

Stomping your foot sends a wave of vibration from the bottom of your foot all the way up your leg and into your body. Pause for a moment after each stomp. Suggest to yourself that you can feel this vibration and trace the pathway as it travels up your leg. Simply play the game that you can see and feel the vibration moving upward. It is happening, and in time you will actually be able to feel it!

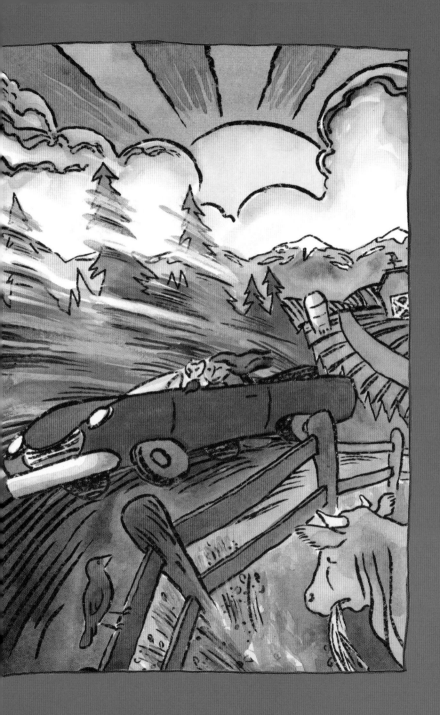

Using Imagery for Better Balance

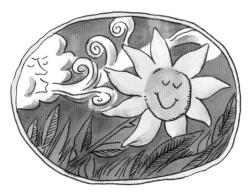

Now that you have wiped away stress and tension, take a moment to enjoy the smooth and unrestricted flow of energy coursing through your body. You have learned that a healthy body depends on good blood flow and circulation, and you have learned massage techniques to make that happen!

Feel free to perform any or all of your Qi massage routine throughout the day. For best results, do the routine 3-5 times each week. You should notice a difference in about two weeks. With regular practice, you will feel relaxed, alert, and more aware of your body. You will be able to move more easily and experience less pain. Although you can't really feel it, your Qi massage routine will boost your immune system and help you fight off colds, flu, and other illness.

Give yourself a pat on the back and be proud that you have decided to live a healthier life! Qi massage can't cure all ills, but now you have the tools to help you live a lifetime filled with energy and harmony.

Your hands are your tools during massage. Becoming an expert with a tool takes practice. For example, using a hammer to pound a nail is awkward at first, but in time becomes second nature. You eventually begin to feel the nail through the hammer itself and learn to apply the appropriate amount of force.

A telephone is also a tool. It helps us communicate across distance. I would like you to imagine that your hands are like a telephone. To be an effective masseur, you need to learn how to send and receive information through your hands just like you use a telephone to talk and listen to your friend. You are both ACTIVE (talking) and RECEPTIVE (listening).

Listening skills are always harder to learn, especially when you are trying to learn how to "listen" with your hands instead of your ears!

The New Forest 1-10 imagery was created by John Bright-Fey to help Tai Chi and meditation students focus mind and body on coordinated, regenerative physical activity. When your body and mind work together as they should, you enter The New Forest. I have applied his system to massage. The New Forest 1 through 10 imagery provides you with a kind of vocabulary so you can communicate with your bodymind and transform your massage skills from mechanical to intuitive.

Start by reading the following list aloud several times.

NUMBER	KEYWORD
1	FUN
2	SHOE
3	TREE
4	CORE
5	ALIVE
6	THICK
7	HEAVEN
8	GATE
9	SHINE
10	SPIN

Now, close your eyes and count from one through ten, saying the numbers and keywords from memory. Recite silently or aloud; you choose. If you get stuck, open your eyes and read the list again until you know all of the keywords and their associated numbers. It won't be long before you have them easily memorized. Each keyword provides a concept and bodymind skill that will improve your massage technique.

1-FUN is your cue to stay relaxed and avoid tensing your muscles. Perform your massage techniques using as little effort as possible. Keep a light smile on your face to generate a sense of relaxation throughout your whole body. Massage should be fun and enjoyable.

QUESTION: Do I feel relaxed?

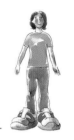

2-SHOE is designed to bring your attention away from your brain and move it down to your feet. Massage is a way for you to connect with your feeling body instead of your thinking mind. When you find yourself thinking too much, gently stomp your feet on the floor. Feel your feet connecting to the earth and ground yourself to the planet.

QUESTION: Can I feel the floor through the bottoms of my feet?

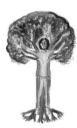

3-TREE imagery reminds you that you are like a tree with deep roots. You gain sustenance and nourishment from the earth. As you perform your massage techniques, remind yourself that you are a living, breathing creature of the earth. Draw nourishment from your roots and transport it through your hands into your body.

QUESTION: Do I feel rooted to the earth like a big tree?

4-CORE is your physical and energetic center. Your center is located near your navel, but a little bit lower and deep inside you. Developing an awareness of your 4-CORE will bring confidence to your movements and provide a sense of stability. Massaging with confidence is necessary to promote health and well-being.

QUESTION: Can I feel my center deep inside my belly?

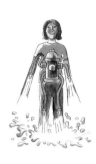

5-ALIVE teaches you gentle strength. Gentle strength comes from deep inside of you. In fact, it comes from your 4-CORE fire hydrant and flows out to your arms and legs! The strength of your touch comes from inside. Learn to feel your internal strength being expressed outward without muscular effort.

QUESTION: Can I feel the subtle strength flowing out of my hands?

6-THICK is designed to connect you to your surroundings. Imagine that the air around you is thick, like water in a swimming pool. As you perform your massage, you are stirring the air, creating swirls of energy around you. Pretend that the thick air that swirls around you soothes your skin.

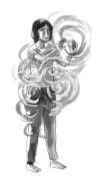

QUESTION: Can I feel the thick air swirling around me?

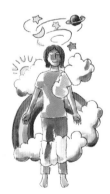

7-HEAVEN connects you to what is above. Stretch up with the crown of your head and your posture naturally improves. Hunching over traps energy and limits circulation. As you perform your massaging movements, think about your goals and aspirations. Connect to your higher ideals and imagine you can be anything you choose.

QUESTION: Do I have a clear idea of my goals and dreams?

8-GATE is your reminder to pay attention to your breathing. To keep your breath relaxed and unrestricted, imagine that each pore of your skin is a tiny gate. As you inhale, these gates swing open and you absorb air and energy. As you exhale, the gates close and the air-energy circulates throughout your entire body. Suggest to yourself that you are breathing with your skin. Breath is important to massage because it promotes circulation.

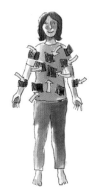

QUESTION: Am I taking full, deep breaths?

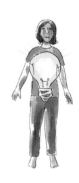

9-SHINE is designed to help you cultivate a positive mental attitude and learn how to exert your energy evenly in all directions. Imagine that you are a light bulb. As you breathe out, your light shines brighter, brighter, brighter! As you breathe in, your light gets dim, dimmer, dimmer. Pretend that you can feel your light shining out in all directions.

QUESTION: Do I have a positive attitude about massaging my body?

10-SPIN teaches you to stay physically and mentally flexible. As you perform your massaging movements, remember to stay open to the messages you bodymind is sending. Randomly cycle through the numbers and images of your New Forest vocabulary. This will help you tune in to your intuition and follow the path to health.

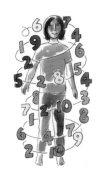

QUESTION: Am I giving myself permission to be open to my intuition?

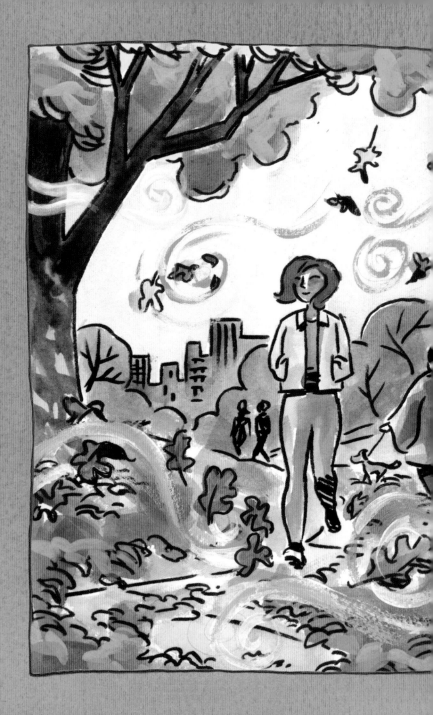

An Extra Sip:

Qi Massage with a Partner

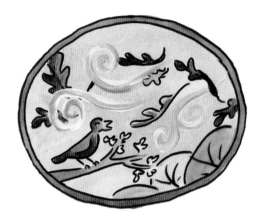

Sharing a massage is a wonderful experience. It is a gift from your heart and your hands. Don't worry about doing it wrong. Simply follow the routine as outlined, and with a little practice, you will feel confident and comfortable. Who knows? Someone might even tell you that your hands are magic!

Prepare the Space

Massage should be performed in a peaceful and comfortable environment. For best results, take the time to prepare your massage setting. Follow these tips:

- Play soft, soothing music.
- Dim the lights and light candles.
- Take the chill out of the room by turning up the heat.
- Turn off the ringer on the phone.

Gather your supplies.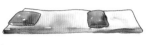

You will need:

- One or two thick, soft blankets
  for your partner to lie upon
  Use extra if you have hard floors
- Two or three pillows

Prepare Yourself

Wear loose comfortable clothing so you can move freely.
Remove your watch, rings, or jewelry that might get in your way.
Take a moment to recite your New Forest massage vocabulary,
silently or aloud. Let the images of each word wash over you and
through you. This will help release unwanted tension and help you
feel relaxed and centered.

Prepare Your Partner

Because Qi massage focuses on the body's energy pathways, or
meridians, your partner can remain fully clothed during the
massage. However, the routine ends with a foot rub, so it is best if
your partner is barefoot. It is important for your partner to feel
comfortable. Ask for feedback during the massage. Some questions
you might ask include the following:

- Are you warm enough?
- Am I using too much/too little pressure?
- Does this feel OK?

Your partner should tell you if:

- Anything you do is painful or unpleasant
- He/She needs a break for any reason

For best results, each of you should concentrate on the massage
itself and avoid unnecessary conversation.

Part One: Activate and Stimulate

Lead your partner through the full body rub found on pages 22-27.

This 2-3 minute routine prepares you and your partner for the massage. See yourself as a conductor preparing the orchestra. Use a clear, calm, and patient voice as you direct your partner from one technique to the next. Stand side by side, or facing each other, while you both activate each part of your body.

- Clap and rub your hands together.
- Activate your arms.
- Activate your back.
- Activate your legs .
- Activate your belly.
- Activate your head and scalp.

Now you are ready to give your partner a Qi massage.

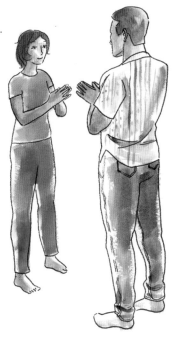

Part Two: Refine and Tonify

Have your partner lie on her back on the soft blankets that you provided. Place a pillow under her knees and under her head. Instruct her to make herself as comfortable as possible. Position yourself near the top of her head. Your comfort is important, so experiment to find a position that works best for you. For more in-depth information about each massage, refer back to the self-massage routine.

MASSAGE THE HEAD
Scalp Massage

Use the pads of your fingers to massage the scalp as if you were washing your partner's hair. Get all over! Don't miss a spot. Be gentle but firm.

Circle the Eye

Use the pads of your first and second fingers to gently circle around the eyes. Use a light touch and skim the surface of the skin. Remember to stay on the bony part that surrounds the eye. Repeat 5-10 times.

Nasal Flare Press

Place the pads of your thumbs at the bottom of your partner's nasal flare. Gently press and massage without lifting your thumbs for 10-15 seconds.

Corner of the Eye

Place the pads of your thumbs at the outside corner of your partner's eye. Stay on the bony part and avoid the temple. Gently press and massage without lifting your thumbs for 10-15 seconds.

Jaw Hinge

Place the pads of your fingers on the thick jaw muscles just below the jaw hinge. Press and massage using gentle but firm pressure for 10-15 seconds.

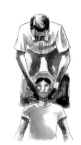

Neck to Shoulder Glide

Start near your partner's head. Use your thumbs to make a long gliding stroke along the sides of the neck to the top of the shoulders. Repeat 5-10 times.

MASSAGE THE BELLY

Position yourself next to your partner's abdomen. Remember to use a light and gentle touch and ask your partner for feedback.

- Make one large circle around the abdomen. Repeat 5-10 times.

- Starting in the center with both hands side by side, make two circles around the abdomen, in opposite directions. Repeat 5-10 times.

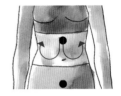

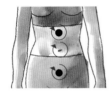

- Make three small clockwise circles along the center line. Repeat 5-10 times.

Massage the Hands

Adjust your position so you can comfortably massage your partner's hand. Perform the entire routine on one hand and then repeat on the other side.

Hand Rub

Take your partner's hand between both of yours. Use one of your hands to support and your other to rub all over your partner's hand. Change the positioning of your hands as needed. Continue for 10-15 seconds.

Center of Palm

Supporting your partner's hand, place the pad of your thumb in the center of your partner's palm. As your partner inhales, gently maintain your position. As your partner exhales, press inward gently and massage. Repeat for 3-5 breaths.

Tiger's Mouth

Supporting your partner's hand, place the pad of your thumb in the Tiger's Mouth area of your partner's hand. As your partner inhales, gently maintain your position. As your partner exhales, press inward gently and massage. Repeat for 3-5 breaths.

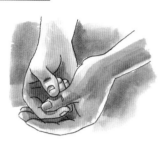

Knuckle Wiggle

Perform the knuckle wiggling sequence found on pages 44-45. Remember to be gentle and ask your partner for feedback. Start at your partner's thumb and work your way to the pinky finger.

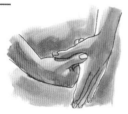

MASSAGE THE FEET

Adjust your position so you can comfortably massage your partner's feet. Perform the entire routine on one foot and then repeat on the other side.

Foot Rub

Take your partner's foot between both of your hands. Use one of your hands to support and your other to rub all over your partner's foot. Change the positioning of your hands as needed. Continue for 10-15 seconds.

Center of Foot

Supporting your partner's foot, place the pad of your thumb in the center of your partner's foot. As your partner inhales, gently maintain your position. As your partner exhales, press inward gently and massage. Repeat for 3-5 breaths.

Heel Massage

Supporting your partner's foot, cup the heel with your palm. Massage the entire heel by gently squeezing and releasing; squeezing and twisting. Continue for 10-15 seconds.

Knuckle Wiggle

Perform the knuckle wiggling sequence found on page 53. Remember to be gentle and ask your partner for feedback. Start at your partner's first toe and work your way to the pinky toe.

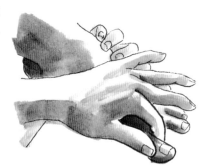

MASSAGE THE BACK

Have your partner roll over to lie face down. Place a pillow under her head and under her ankles. Another pillow can be used under her hips if needed to reduce strain on the low back.

Pressing Spots

Place the pad of your first finger and thumb on the muscles that run directly next to the spine. Start at the base of the neck. Gently press down and wiggle your fingers a bit. Lift and move down about 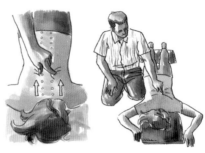 one inch. Press and wiggle again. Lift and move down another inch. Press and wiggle. Work your way down the full length of the spine, inch by inch. Repeat 1-3 times.

Extra Attention

- Use equal pressure under your index finger and thumb.
- Avoid pressing directly on the bony spine. Stay on the muscles.
- Use the pads of your fingers so that you don't poke your partner with your fingernails. Remember to ask for feedback and adjust your pressure accordingly.

Long Strokes

Place your hands at the base of your partner's neck. Using one long gliding motion, stroke gently down the full length of the spine. Repeat 5-10 times.

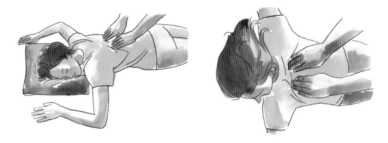

Extra Attention

- Use equal pressure under both hands.
- Experiment with the speed of your stroke. Ask your partner which feels best. Slow? Medium? Fast?
- Stroke the muscles, not the spine.

ENDING THE ROUTINE

Cover your partner with a light blanket to keep her warm and relaxed. Tell her that the massage has come to an end using a soft and soothing voice. Instruct her to remain lying down as long as she likes and to take her time getting up.

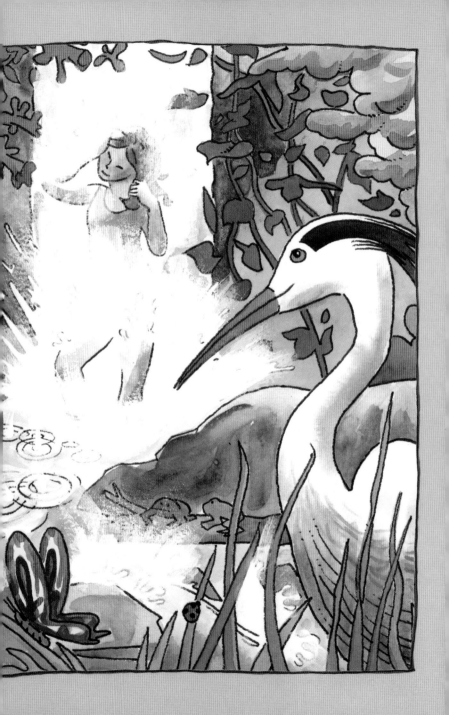

If you would like to learn more about...

MASSAGE:
American Massage Therapy Association
www.amtamassage.org

American Physical Therapy Association
www.apta.org

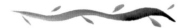

ASIAN-BASED MASSAGE AND TRADITIONAL CHINESE MEDICINE
www.qi-journal.com

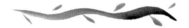

BOOKS AND DVDS BY KIM BRIGHT-FEY:

1. *A Morning Cup of Massage:* one 15-minute routine for a lifetime of energy & harmony

2. New Forest Tai Chi for Beginners DVD
   UPC: 827912001556

The Morning Cup™ Series

To improve your balance, try:

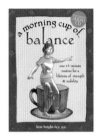 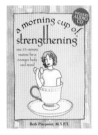 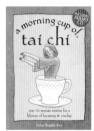 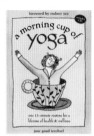

To increase your strengthening and flexibility:

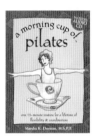 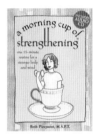 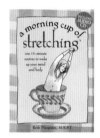

To increase your energy and well-being:

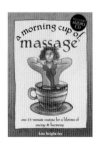 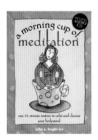 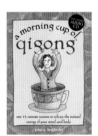 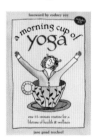

About the Author

Kim Bright-Fey is a licensed physical therapist who is certified with the American Physical Therapy Association as a health and wellness consultant. She has been teaching Qigong, Tai Chi, and therapeutic exercise since 1988. She lives in Birmingham, Alabama.

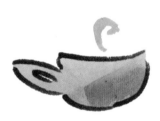

Routine at a Glance

PART ONE: ACTIVATE AND STIMULATE

Activate Your Hands

Activate Your Arms

Activate Your Back

Activate Your Legs

Activate Your Belly

Activate Your Head and Scalp

Finishing the Full Body Rub

PART TWO: REFINE AND TONIFY

HEAD MASSAGE

Pound Your Neck

Circling the Eye

Nasal Flare

Corner Of Eye

Sinus Massage

Jaw Hinge

Head Drumming

Head Rub

ABDOMEN MASSAGE

Belly Circle 1

Belly Circle 2

Belly Circle 3

HAND MASSAGE

Activate Your Hands

Center of Palm

Tiger's Mouth

Knuckle Wiggle

Open - Close Hands

Thumb Hold

FOOT MASSAGE

Activate Your Hands and Feet

Center of Foot

Heel Massage

Knuckle Wiggle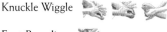

Foot Pounding

Point and Flex

Foot Stomp

Tear this page out and post it on your refrigerator or another handy spot for quick reference to your massage routine.